MW00510217

The Essential Instant Pot Cookbook for Beginners

Quick And Easy Delicious Dishes To Prepare At Home

Irma Dobson

© Copyright 2021 - All rights reserved.

The content contained within this book may not be reproduced, duplicated or transmitted without direct written permission from the author or the publisher.

Under no circumstances will any blame or legal responsibility be held against the publisher, or author, for any damages, reparation, or monetary loss due to the information contained within this book. Either directly or indirectly.

Legal Notice:

This book is copyright protected. This book is only for personal use. You cannot amend, distribute, sell, use, quote or paraphrase any part, or the content within this book, without the consent of the author or publisher.

Disclaimer Notice:

Please note the information contained within this document is for educational and entertainment purposes only. All effort has been executed to present accurate, up to date, and reliable, complete information. No warranties of any kind are declared or implied. Readers acknowledge that the author is not engaging in the rendering of legal, financial, medical or professional advice. The content within this book has been derived from various sources. Please consult a licensed professional before attempting any techniques outlined in this book.

By reading this document, the reader agrees that under no circumstances is the author responsible for any losses, direct or indirect, which are incurred as a result of the use of information contained within this document, including, but not limited to, — errors, omissions, or inaccuracies.

Sommario

Introduction 7

Side Dishes 9

   Peppery Bok Choy 9

   Artichoke with Creamy Sauce 11

   Kabocha Ginger Squash 13

   Thai Zucchini Strips 15

   Paprika Carrots 18

   Healthy Turnip-Broccoli Mash 21

   Sautéed Pineapple 23

   Enoki Mix 25

   Bell Cabbage Wedges 27

   Pepper Celery Stalk 30

   Provolone Mac&Cheese 32

   Mushrooms Casserole 35

   Butter Mushrooms 37

   Bacon and Leek 39

   Provolone Mash with Bacon 41

   Butter Cauliflower 43

   Nutmeg Cauliflower Slices 45

   Onion Mashed Brussel Sprouts 48

   Chicken Cauliflower Rice 50

   Soft Spinach with Dill 52

   Mexican Rice 54

   Pecans Parmesan Bowl 56

Cabbage in Cream 58

Dill Cheese 61

Cauliflower-Tatoes 63

Salty Spaghetti Squash 65

Mozzarella Zucchini Casserole 67

Button Beans Casserole 69

Ground Zucchini Casserole 71

Almons and Mozzarella Zucchini Strips 73

Cabbage Rice 76

Cheddar Creamy Gratin 78

White Onion Rings 80

Rosemary Halves 82

Sweet Baby Carrot 84

Chili Zucchini Bowl 86

Thyme Asparagus 89

Minced Radish 91

Peppery Cubes 93

Pecan Salad 95

Cheese Gnocchi 97

Purple Cabbage Steaks 100

Cauliflower and Goat Cheese 103

Mushrooms and Fall Vegetables 105

Garlic Broccoli 107

Tots with Broccoli 109

Vegetable Fritters 111

Pressured Asparagus 113

Roasted Cider Steak...115

Cayenne Pepper Green Beans......................................117

Conclusion..119

Introduction

This complete and valuable overview to immediate pot cooking with over 1000 dishes for morning meal, supper, supper, as well as even treats! This is among the most comprehensive split second pot cookbooks ever before released thanks to its selection as well as exact directions. Innovative dishes and also classics, modern-day take on family's most loved meals-- all this is tasty, straightforward and also obviously as healthy and balanced as it can be. Adjustment the means you cook with these cutting-edge immediate pot instructions. Required a new supper or a dessert? Below you are! Best instant pot dishes come together in a few straightforward actions, also a beginner can do it! The instant pot specifies the means you prepare every day. This instant pot cookbook aids you make the outright most out of your once a week menu. The only split second pot book you will ever before need with the utmost collection of recipes will assist you towards an easier and also healthier kitchen area experience. If you wish to save time cooking meals much more effectively, if you want to use your household food that can satisfy also the pickiest eater, you remain in the ideal location! Master your split second pot as well as make your food preparation requires match your hectic way of living.

Side Dishes

Peppery Bok Choy

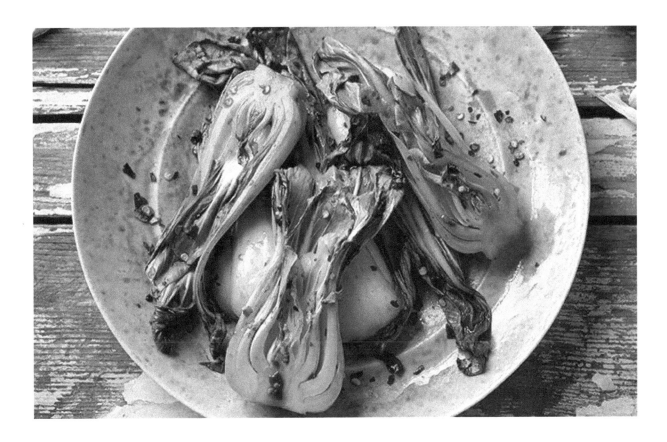

Prep time: 10 minutes

Cooking time: 8 minutes

Servings: 2

Ingredients:

- 9 oz bok choy

- 1 tablespoon olive oil

- 1 teaspoon lemon juice

- 1 teaspoon ground black pepper

Directions:

1. Wash and trim the bok choy. Cut the vegetables into halves and sprinkle with lemon juice. Transfer them in the cooker. Add olive oil and ground black pepper. Mix up the vegetables with the help of the wooden spatula.

2. Set air crisp mode and close the lid. Cook the vegetables for 8 minutes. Stir them after 4 minutes of cooking. The cooked bok choy should have a tender texture.

Nutrition: calories 77, fat 7.3, fiber 1.3, carbs 2.8, protein 1.9

Artichoke with Creamy Sauce

Prep time: 8 minutes

Cooking time: 8 minutes

Servings: 5

Ingredients:

- 1-pound artichoke petals

- 1 cup heavy cream

- 3 oz Cheddar cheese, shredded

- 1 teaspoon minced garlic

- 1 teaspoon garlic powder

- 1 teaspoon chili flakes

- 1 teaspoon almond flour

- 1 tablespoon butter

- ½ teaspoon salt

Directions:

1. Mix up together artichoke petals, minced garlic, garlic powder, and chili flakes. Add salt. Transfer the mixture in the cooker.

2. Add shredded cheese, almond flour, and cream. Mix it up. Close and seal the lid. Cook the side dish for 8 minutes on High-pressure mode.

3. Then use quick pressure release and open the lid.

4. Mix up the artichoke petals with sauce gently and transfer into the serving bowls.

Nutrition: calories 220, fat 17.2, fiber 5, carbs 11.1, protein 7.9

Kabocha Ginger Squash

Prep time: 10 minutes

Cooking time: 2 hours

Servings: 2

Ingredients:

- 1 ½ cup kabocha squash, chopped

- ½ teaspoon ground cinnamon

- ½ teaspoon Erythritol

- 1 tablespoon butter

- ½ teaspoon ground ginger

- ½ cup of water

Directions:

1. In the cooker, mix up together kabocha squash, ground cinnamon, ginger, and Erythritol. Add butter and water.

2. Close and seal the lid.

3. Cook the vegetable on Low-pressure mode for 2 hours.

4. When the time is over and the squash is tender, transfer it in the serving bowl, add gravy from the cooker and serve.

Nutrition: calories 84, fat 5.8, fiber 1.4, carbs 7.8, protein 1.1

Thai Zucchini Strips

Prep time: 10 minutes

Cooking time: 15 minutes

Servings: 8

Ingredients:

- 3 medium green zucchini

- 1 teaspoon ground black pepper

- ½ cup of soy sauce

- 1 tablespoon sesame seeds

- 1 teaspoon salt

- ½ tablespoon Erythritol

- 1 tablespoon butter

- 1 tablespoon heavy cream

- 1 teaspoon cilantro

- 1 egg

- 1 teaspoon cumin seeds

- ½ cup almond flour

Directions:

1. Wash the zucchini and cut it into the strips.

2. Combine the ground black pepper, sesame seeds, salt, and cilantro together in a mixing bowl. Add cumin seeds.

3. Combine Erythritol and soy sauce and blend. Add the egg to the mixing bowl and whisk. Sprinkle the zucchini strips with the whisked egg.

4. Blend the mixture well using your hands. Sprinkle the zucchini strips with the almond flour, then sprinkle the zucchini with the ground black pepper mixture.

5. Add the butter to the pressure cooker and add the cream. Add the zucchini strips. Make the layer from the zucchini strips.

6. Cook the zucchini on the "Pressure" mode for 5 minutes. Remove and add a second layer of zucchini. Repeat this until all the zucchini are cooked.

7. Put the cooked zucchini strips in the pressure cooker.

8. Add the soy sauce mixture. Close the lid and sauté the dish for 3 minutes.

9. When the cooking time ends, transfer the dish to serving plates.

Nutrition: calories 61, fat 4.2, fiber 1.3, carbs 3.7, protein 2.8

Paprika Carrots

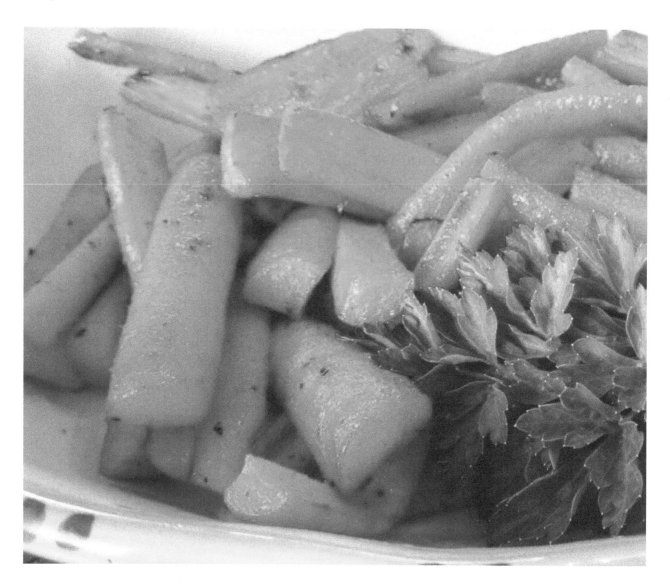

Prep time: 10 minutes

Cooking time: 10 minutes

Servings: 8

Ingredients:

- 1 pound carrots

- 9 ounces sliced bacon

- 1 teaspoon salt

- ½ teaspoon ground black pepper

- 1 teaspoon ground white pepper

- 1 teaspoon paprika

- ¼ cup chicken stock

- 1 tablespoon olive oil

- ¼ teaspoon marjoram

Directions:

1. Wash the carrot and peel it. Sprinkle the carrot with the ground black pepper.

2. Combine the salt, ground white pepper, paprika, and marjoram and stir the mixture. Coat the sliced bacon with the spice mixture.

3. Wrap the carrots in the sliced bacon. Pour the olive oil in the pressure cooker and add wrapped carrots.

4. Close the lid, set the pressure cooker to "Sauté" mode, and sauté the carrot for 10 minutes.

5. Add the chicken stock and cook the dish on the pressure mode for 8 minutes.

6. When the cooking time ends, release the pressure and open the lid. Serve warm.

Nutrition: calories 141, fat 11.4, fiber 3, carbs 7.91, protein 4

Healthy Turnip-Broccoli Mash

Prep time: 15 minutes

Cooking time: 25 minutes

Servings: 6

Ingredients:

- 8 ounces turnip

- 5 ounces broccoli

- 2 cups chicken stock

- ¼ cup cream

- 1 tablespoon salt

- 1 teaspoon cilantro

- 2 tablespoons butter

- ⅓ teaspoon thyme

Directions:

1. Peel the turnip and cut the broccoli into florets.

2. Chop the turnip and broccoli florets and place them in the pressure cooker. Add salt, cilantro, and butter and blend well.

3. Add chicken stock and close the lid. Set the pressure cooker to "Steam" mode and cook for 25 minutes.

4. When the cooking time ends, remove the vegetables from the pressure cooker. Leave a ½ cup of the liquid from the cooked vegetables.

5. Place the vegetables in a blender. Add the vegetable liquid and cream. Puree the mixture until smooth.

6. Add the butter and blend it for 2 minutes. Serve the potato-broccoli mash warm.

Nutrition: calories 62, fat 4.7, fiber 1.3, carbs 4.6, protein 1.4

Sautéed Pineapple

Prep time: 5 minutes

Cooking time: 10 minutes

Servings: 5

Ingredients:

- 9 ounces pineapple

- 1 tablespoon Erythritol

- ¼ cup lemon juice

- 3 tablespoons water

- 1 teaspoon cinnamon

- 1 teaspoon peanut oil

- ½ teaspoon paprika

Directions:

1. Peel the pineapple and cut it into the cubes.

2. Put the peanut oil in the pressure cooker. Add pineapple cubes, set the pressure cooker to "Sauté" mode, and sauté the fruit for 3 minutes, stirring frequently.

3. Add Erythritol, lemon juice, water, cinnamon, and paprika.

4. Blend the mixture gently. Close the lid and sauté the pineapple mixture for 7 minutes.

5. When the cooking time ends, remove the pineapple with the liquid from the pressure cooker. Serve it warm or chilled.

Nutrition: calories 38, fat 1.1, fiber 1.1, carbs 7.5, protein 0.4

Enoki Mix

Prep time: 10 minutes

Cooking time: 9 minutes

Servings: 4

Ingredients:

- 1-pound Enoki mushrooms

- 1 teaspoon salt

- 1 teaspoon sesame seeds

- 1 tablespoon canola oil

- 1 tablespoon apple cider vinegar

- 1 teaspoon paprika

- 1 tablespoon butter

- ½ teaspoon lemon zest

- 1 cup water for cooking

Directions:

1. Slice the mushrooms roughly and place in the cooker. Add water and salt.

2. Close and seal the lid. Cook the vegetables on High-pressure mode for 9 minutes.

3. Then allow natural pressure release. Open the lid and drain the water.

4. Transfer the mushrooms in the bowl.

5. Sprinkle them with the sesame seeds, canola oil, apple cider vinegar, paprika, butter, and lemon zest. Mix up well.

Nutrition: calories 113, fat 7.2, fiber 3.4, carbs 9.3, protein 3.2

Bell Cabbage Wedges

Prep time: 10 minutes

Cooking time: 25 minutes

Servings: 8

Ingredients:

- 10 ounces cabbage
- 3 tablespoons tomato paste
- 1 cup chicken stock
- 1 teaspoon butter
- 1 sweet bell pepper
- ¼ cup sour cream
- 1 teaspoon cilantro
- 1 teaspoon basil
- 1 medium yellow onion

Directions:

1. Wash the cabbage and cut it into the wedges. Place the cabbage wedges into the pressure cooker.

2. Combine the chicken stock, butter, tomato paste, sour cream, cilantro, and basil together in a mixing bowl and blend until smooth.

3. Peel the onion and remove seeds from the bell pepper. Chop the vegetables.

4. Add the chopped vegetables in the cabbage wedges mixture. Add chicken stock sauce and mix well using a wooden spoon or spatula.

5. Close the pressure cooker lid and cook the dish on "Pressure" mode for 25 minutes.

6. When the cooking time ends, open the pressure cooker lid and let the mixture rest briefly. Do not stir it. Transfer the dish to serving plates.

Nutrition: calories 45, fat 2.2, fiber 1.6, carbs 6, protein 1.3

Pepper Celery Stalk

Prep time: 10 minutes

Cooking time: 3 minutes

Servings: 4

Ingredients:

- 1-pound celery stalk

- 1 oz pork rind

- 1 teaspoon ground black pepper

- 1 teaspoon olive oil

- 1 teaspoon salt

- 1 cup water, for cooking

Directions:

1. Chop the celery stalk roughly and place it in the pressure cooker.

2. Add water, close and seal the lid. Cook it on High-pressure mode for 3 minutes. Then allow natural pressure release and open the lid.

3. Drain water and transfer celery stalk in the bowl.

4. Add ground black pepper, olive oil, salt, and pork rind. Mix up the ingredients well and transfer in the serving bowl (plates).

Nutrition: calories 70, fat 3.94, fiber 2, carbs 3.7, protein 5.4

Provolone Mac&Cheese

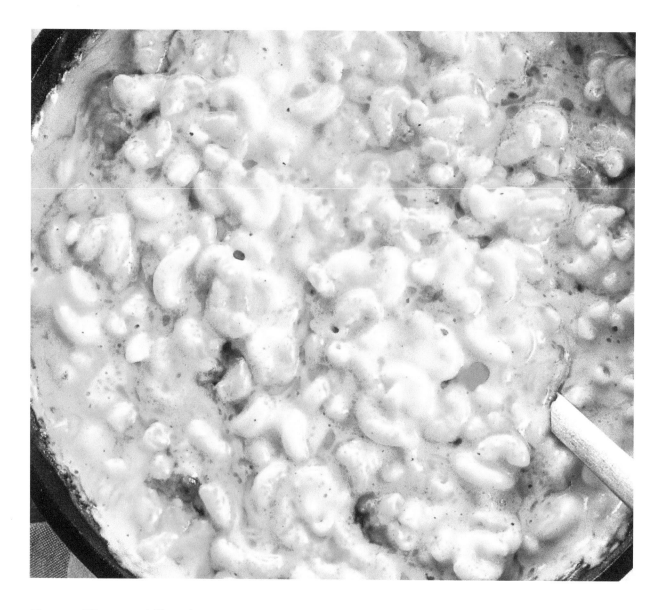

Prep time: 15 minutes

Cooking time: 5 minutes

Servings: 4

Ingredients:

- 2 cups cauliflower, shredded

- ½ cup Provolone cheese, grated

- 1 tablespoon cream cheese

- ¼ cup of coconut milk

- ¼ teaspoon salt

- ½ teaspoon white pepper

Directions:

1. Put shredded cauliflower in the instant pot bowl.

2. Top it with Provolone cheese.

3. After this, in the mixing bowl combine together cream cheese, coconut milk, salt, and white pepper.

4. Pour the liquid over the cheese and close the lid.

5. Cook the side dish on manual mode (high pressure) for 5 minutes.

6. When the time is over, allow the natural pressure release for 5 minutes more.

7. Broil the surface of the cooked meal with the help of the kitchen torch.

Nutrition value/serving: calories 114, fat 8.9, fiber 1.7, carbs 4.1, protein 5.8

Mushrooms Casserole

Prep time: 10 minutes

Cooking time: 4 hours

Ingredients:

- 1 cup Brussels sprouts, halved

- ½ cup heavy cream

- ½ teaspoon ground black pepper

- ½ cup mushrooms, sliced

- 1 teaspoon salt

- 1 oz Monterey Jack cheese, shredded

Directions:

1. In the mixing bowl combine together cheese with heavy cream, salt, and ground black pepper.

2. Place the Brussel sprouts in the instant pot in one layer.

3. Then top it with sliced mushrooms.

4. Pour the heavy cream mixture over the mushrooms and close the lid.

5. Cook the casserole on manual mode (low pressure) for 4 hours.

Nutrition value/serving: calories 120, fat 10.4, fiber 1.3, carbs 3.9, protein 4.1

Butter Mushrooms

Prep time: 5 minutes

Cooking time: 7 minutes

Servings: 2

Ingredients:

- 8 oz white mushrooms, chopped

- 1 teaspoon dried rosemary

- 2 tablespoons butter

- ½ teaspoon salt

- 1 cup chicken broth

- ¼ cup of coconut milk

- ½ teaspoon dried oregano

Directions:

1. Put mushrooms and butter in the instant pot and cook them on sauté mode for 4 minutes.

2.   Then add chicken broth, dried oregano, salt, and coconut milk

3.   Close the lid and cook the side dish on manual mode (high pressure) for 3 minutes.

4.   When the time is over, make a quick pressure release.

5.   Serve the mushrooms with coconut-butter gravy.

Nutrition value/serving: calories 182, fat 13, fiber 3.4, carbs 9.8, protein 10.2

Bacon and Leek

Prep time: 10 minutes

Cooking time: 10 minutes

Servings: 6

Ingredients:

- 12 oz Brussels sprouts

- 3oz leek, chopped

- 2 oz bacon, chopped

- 1 teaspoon avocado oil

- ½ teaspoon salt

- 1 cup water, for cooking

Directions:

1. Pour water and insert the steamer rack in the instant pot.

2.   Then trim Brussel sprouts and cut them into halves.

3.   Arrange the vegetables in the steamer rack and cook on high pressure for 3 minutes. Then make a quick pressure release.

4.   Remove the Brussel sprouts from the instant pot.

5.   Clean the instant pot and rid of the steamer rack.

6.   Put bacon in the instant pot.

7.   Add avocado oil and cook the ingredients on sauté mode for 4 minutes. Stir them halfway of cooking.

8.   Then add leek and cook the mixture for 2 minutes more.

9.   Add the Brussel sprouts, mix up well and sauté the meal for 1 minute.

Nutrition value/serving: calories 85, fat 4.3, fiber 2.4, carbs 7.3, protein 5.7

Provolone Mash with Bacon

Prep time: 10 minutes

Cooking time: 8 minutes

Servings: 3

Ingredients:

- 1 oz bacon, chopped, cooked

- 1 cup spinach, chopped

- 1 tablespoon cream cheese

- ¼ teaspoon minced garlic

- ¼ cup Provolone cheese, grated

- ¼ cup heavy cream

- ¼ cup onion, diced

- ½ teaspoon white pepper

- 1 teaspoon cayenne pepper

- ½ teaspoon salt

- 1 cup water, for cooking

Directions:

1. Put all ingredients in the instant pot baking pan.

2. Pour water and insert the trivet in the instant pot.

3. Place the baking pan with spinach mixture in the instant pot.

4. Cook the dip on manual (high pressure) 8 minutes.

5. When the time is over, allow the natural pressure release for 10 minutes and open the lid.

6. Mix up the spinach mash carefully with the help of the spoon.

Nutrition value/serving: calories 145, fat 11.9, fiber 0.7, carbs 2.7, protein 7.3

Butter Cauliflower

Prep time: 10 minutes

Cooking time: 4 minutes

Servings: 1

Ingredients:

- 1 cup cauliflower, chopped

- ¼ teaspoon salt

- 1 tablespoon butter

- 1 cup water, for cooking

Directions:

1. Pour water and insert the steamer rack in the instant pot.

2. Place the chopped cauliflower on the rack and close the lid.

3. Cook the vegetables for 4 minutes on Steam mode. When the time is over, make a quick pressure release.

4. Transfer the cooked cauliflower in the bowl. Add butter and salt.

5. With the help of the potato masher mash the vegetables until smooth.

6. Add ¼ cup of water from the instant pot. If the mash is not soft enough – add more water.

7. Mix up the mashed cauliflower well.

Nutrition value/serving: calories 127, fat 11.6, fiber 2.5, carbs 5.3, protein 2.1

Nutmeg Cauliflower Slices

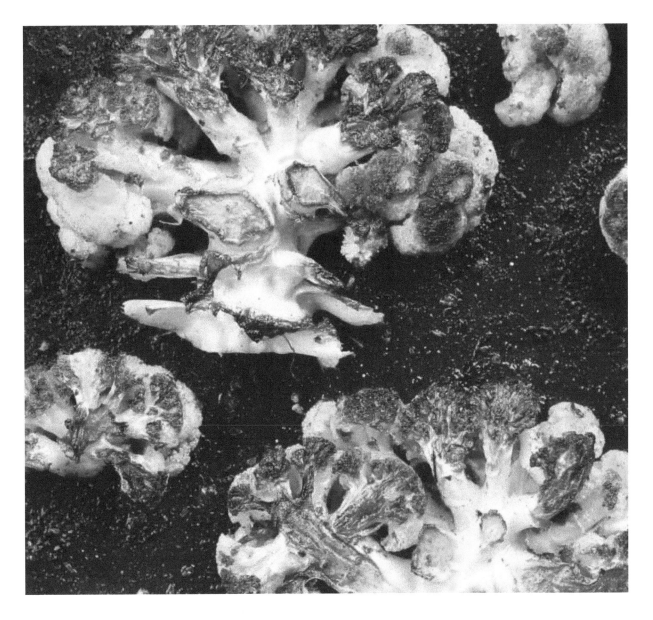

Prep time: 10 minutes

Cooking time: 5 minutes

Servings: 3

Ingredients:

- 9 oz cauliflower head, trimmed

- 1 teaspoon ground nutmeg

- ½ teaspoon ground paprika

- ½ teaspoon ground turmeric

- ½ teaspoon dried oregano

- 1 tablespoon lemon juice

- 1 tablespoon avocado oil

- ¼ teaspoon minced garlic

- 1 tablespoon heavy cream

- 1 cup water, for cooking

Directions:

1. Slice the cauliflower into the steaks.

2. Then pour water in the instant pot. Insert the steamer rack.

3. Place the cauliflower steaks on the rack and close the lid.

4. Cook the vegetables on manual mode (high pressure) for 2 minutes. Then make a quick pressure release.

5. Remove the cauliflower steaks and clean the instant pot.

6. In the shallow bowl combine together ground nutmeg, paprika, turmeric, oregano, lemon juice, avocado oil, minced garlic, and heavy cream.

7. Carefully brush the cauliflower slices with spice mixture from both side and place in the instant pot in one layer.

8. Cook the cauliflower on sauté mode for 1 minute from each side or until it light brown.

9. Repeat the same steps with remaining cauliflower slices.

Nutrition value/serving: calories 53, fat 3, fiber 2.8, carbs 6.1, protein 2

Onion Mashed Brussel Sprouts

Prep time: 10 minutes

Cooking time: 5 minutes

Servings: 4

Ingredients:

- 2 cups Brussel sprouts

- ½ teaspoon onion powder

- ¼ cup heavy cream, hot

- ¼ teaspoon salt

- 1 cup water, for cooking

Directions:

1. Pour water and insert the steamer rack in the instant pot.

2. Place the Brussel sprouts in the rack and cook it on manual mode (high pressure) for 5 minutes.

3.   When the time is over, make a quick pressure release.

4.   Transfer the cooked vegetables in the food processor.

5.   Add cream, salt, and onion powder.

6.   Blend the mixture until is smooth.

7.   Put the cooked mashed Brussel sprouts in the bowls.

8.   It is recommended to serve the side dish warm or hot.

Nutrition value/serving: calories 46, fat 2.9, fiber 1.7, carbs 4.5, protein 1.7

Chicken Cauliflower Rice

Prep time: 2 minutes

Cooking time: 1 minute

Servings: 2

Ingredients:

- 1 cup cauliflower, shredded

- 5 oz chicken broth

Directions:

1. Put cauliflower and chicken broth in the instant pot.

2. Set manual mode (high pressure) and cook cauliflower for 1 minute.

3. Then make a quick pressure release. Add salt and ground black pepper if desired.

Nutrition value/serving: calories 24, fat 0.5, fiber 1.3, carbs 2.9, protein 2.4

Soft Spinach with Dill

Prep time: 5 minutes

Cooking time: 10 minutes

Servings: 2

Ingredients:

- 2 cup fresh spinach, chopped

- 1 teaspoon avocado oil

- 1 tablespoon fresh dill, chopped

- 1 teaspoon lemon juice

- ¼ teaspoon salt

- 1 teaspoon butter

- ¼ teaspoon onion powder

Directions:

1. Set instant pot on sauté mode and adjust 10 minutes.

2. Pour avocado oil and add chopped spinach.

3. Sprinkle the greens with dill, lemon juice, salt, and onion powder.

4. Add butter.

5. Stir the spinach every 2 minutes.

Nutrition value/serving: calories 32, fat 2.4, fiber 1, carbs 2.4, protein 1.3

Mexican Rice

Prep time: 5 minutes

Cooking time: 4 minutes

Servings: 5

Ingredients:

- 3 cups cauliflower, shredded

- ½ teaspoon taco seasonings

- ½ teaspoon garlic powder

- 1 teaspoon lime juice

- 1 teaspoon dried cilantro

- 1 bell pepper, diced

- 2 cups chicken broth

- ½ teaspoon salt

Directions:

1. In the shallow bowl combine together taco seasonings, garlic powder, salt, and dried cilantro.

2. Then put shredded cauliflower in the instant pot bowl.

3. Add spice mixture.

4. After this, add lime juice, bell pepper, and chicken broth.

5. Gently mix up the vegetables with the help of the spoon.

6. Close the lid of the instant pot and cook the meal on manual (high pressure) for 4 minutes.

7. When the time is over, make a quick pressure release.

8. Stir the side dish well.

Nutrition value/serving: calories 42, fat 0.7, fiber 1.9, carbs 6.2, protein 3.4

Pecans Parmesan Bowl

Prep time: 5 minutes

Cooking time: 10 minutes

Servings: 3

Ingredients:

- 3 pecans

- 7 oz curly kale, chopped

- 2 oz Parmesan, grated

- 2 tablespoon cream cheese

Directions:

1. Put the pecans in the grinder and grind until you get smooth mass.

2. Then mix up together grinded pecans with cream cheese.

3.   Heat up the instant pot on sauté mode for 2 minutes.

4.   Add cream cheese mixture and kale.

5.   Cook the ingredients for 4 minutes. Stir them halfway of cooking.

6.   Then add cheese.

7.   Cook the meal for 4 minutes more or until the kale is tender.

Nutrition value/serving: calories 214, fat 17, fiber 3.9, carbs 8.7, protein 10.9

Cabbage in Cream

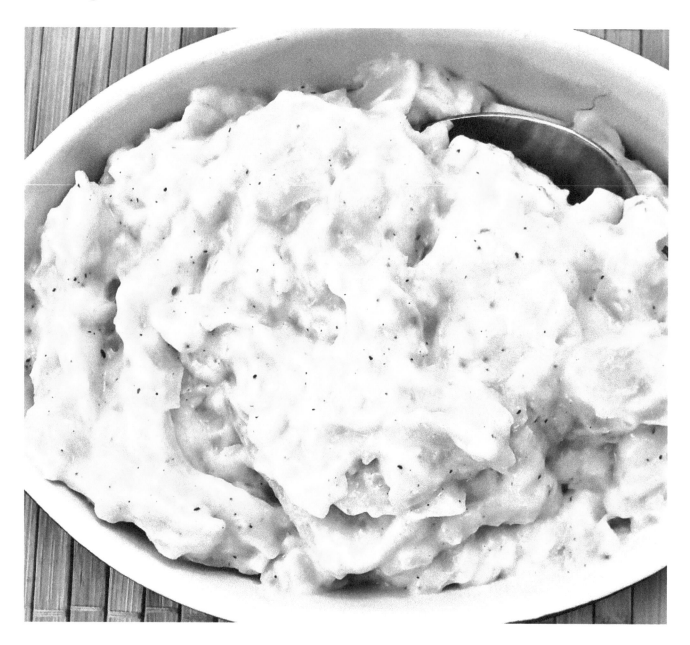

Prep time: 5 minutes

Cooking time: 7 hours

Servings: 4

Ingredients:

- 12 oz white cabbage, roughly chopped

- 1 cup cream

- 1 tablespoon cream cheese

- 1 teaspoon salt

- 1 teaspoon chili powder

Directions:

1. Put all ingredients in the instant pot bowl and close the lid.

2. Cook the vegetables for 7 minutes on manual mode (high pressure).

3. When the time is over, make a quick pressure release.

4. Open the instant pot lid and stir the cooked side dish well.

Nutrition value/serving: calories 71, fat 4.4, fiber 2.4, carbs 7.2, protein 1.8

Dill Cheese

Prep time: 5 minutes

Cooking time: 15 minutes

Servings: 2

Ingredients:

- ½ cup cauliflower, cut into florets

- ½ teaspoon dried dill

- ¼ teaspoon dried cilantro

- ¼ teaspoon dried sage

- 3 oz Parmesan, grated

- ¼ cup of organic almond milk

Directions:

1. Put cauliflower in the instant pot bowl.

2. Sprinkle it with dried dill, cilantro, and sage.

3.   In the separated bowl mix up together almond milk and Parmesan.

4.   Pour the liquid over the cauliflower and close the lid.

5.   Cook the meal on sauté mode for 15 minutes. Stir the cauliflower every 5 minutes to avoid burning.

Nutrition value/serving: calories 164, fat 10.7, fiber 1.2, carbs 4, protein 14.7

Cauliflower-Tatoes

Prep time: 10 minutes

Cooking time: 5 minutes

Servings: 2

Ingredients:

- 1 teaspoon cream cheese

- ½ teaspoon salt

- ½ teaspoon ground turmeric

- ½ teaspoon white pepper

- 2 cups cauliflower

- ½ teaspoon garlic powder

- 1 cup water, for cooking

Directions:

1. Pour water and insert the trivet in the instant pot.

2. Put the cauliflower on the trivet and cook it for 5 minutes on steam mode. Then make a quick pressure release.

3. Open the lid and transfer cooked cauliflower in the food processor.

4. Add salt, ground turmeric, cream cheese, white pepper, and garlic powder.

5. Then add ¾ cup of the remaining water from the instant pot.

6. Blend the mixture until it is smooth (appx for 3-5 minutes).

Nutrition value/serving: calories 36, fat 0.8, fiber 2.8, carbs 6.6, protein 2.3

Salty Spaghetti Squash

Prep time: 10 minutes

Cooking time: 6 minutes

Servings: 3

Ingredients:

- 2 cups spaghetti squash, cubed

- 2 tablespoons butter

- ½ teaspoon salt

- 1 cup water, for cooking

Directions:

1. Pour water and insert the steamer rack in the instant pot.

2. Arrange the spaghetti squash cubes in the instant pot and cook them on manual mode (high pressure) for 6 minutes.

3.   Then make a quick pressure release and open the lid.

4.   Transfer the cooked squash cube sin the serving plates and top them with butter and salt. Wait till butter and salt dissolve.

Nutrition value/serving: calories 89, fat 2, fiber 8.1, carbs 4.7, protein 0.5

Mozzarella Zucchini Casserole

Prep time: 10 minutes

Cooking time: 5 minutes

Servings: 4

Ingredients:

- 2 zucchini, sliced

- 1 tomato, sliced

- ½ cup kohlrabi, chopped

- ½ cup chicken broth

- 1 teaspoon salt

- 1 teaspoon ground paprika

- 1 tablespoon nuts, chopped

- ½ cup Mozzarella, chopped

- ½ teaspoon sesame oil

Directions:

1. Brush the instant pot bowl with sesame oil.

2. Place the zucchini slices in the instant pot.

3. Then top them with sliced tomato and chopped kohlrabi.

4. After this, mix up together chicken broth, salt, and ground paprika.

5. Pour the liquid over the ingredients.

6. Then sprinkle the casserole mixture with nuts and Mozzarella.

7. Close the lid and cook the casserole on High pressure (manual mode) for 5 minutes.

8. When the time is over, make a quick pressure release.

9. Cool the cooked casserole to the room temperature.

Nutrition value/serving: calories 57, fat 2.8, fiber 2.3, carbs 6, protein 3.7

Button Beans Casserole

Prep time: 10 minutes

Cooking time: 20 minutes

Servings: 6

Ingredients:

- 1-pound green beans, chopped

- 1 cup button mushrooms, chopped

- 1 garlic clove, diced

- ½ white onion, diced

- 1 teaspoon butter

- 1/3 cup heavy cream

- ½ teaspoon salt

- 2 tablespoons almond meal

- 1 teaspoon Italian seasonings

- 1 teaspoon coconut oil, melted

Directions:

1.   Toss butter in the instant pot and melt it on sauté mode.

2.   Add onion and cook it for 2 minutes.

3.   Then stir it and add mushrooms.

4.   Cook the mixture for 2 minutes more.

5.   Stir the ingredients again and add garlic clove, green beans, and salt. Mix up well.

6.   In the mixing bowl combine together coconut oil, Italian seasonings, almond meal, and cream.

7.   Pour the liquid over the casserole mixture and close the lid.

8.   Cook it on sauté mode for 16 minutes.

Nutrition value/serving: calories 79, fat 5.2, fiber 3.2, carbs 7.5, protein 2.5

Ground Zucchini Casserole

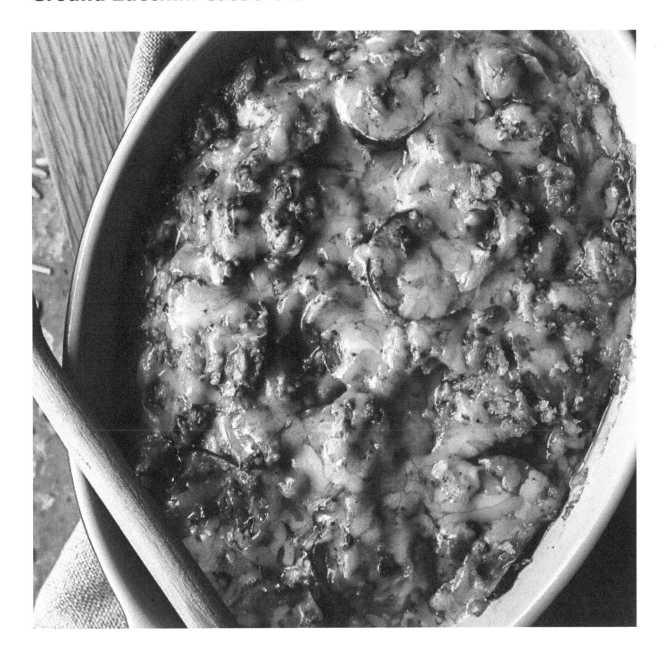

Prep time: 10 minutes

Cooking time: 5 minutes

Servings: 3

Ingredients:

- 7 oz spaghetti squash, chopped

- 1 zucchini, grated

- ½ cup Cheddar cheese

- 1 tablespoon cream cheese

- ½ teaspoon salt

- 1 teaspoon ground black pepper

- 1 cup water, for cooking

Directions:

1. Make the layer of spaghetti squash in the baking pan and top it with grated zucchini.

2. After this, sprinkle the zucchini with Cheddar cheese.

3. In the mixing bowl combine together cream cheese, salt, and ground black pepper.

4. Spread the mixture over the Cheddar cheese.

5. Pour water and insert the trivet in the instant pot.

6. Place the baking pan with casserole in the instant pot and cook it on manual mode (high pressure) for 6 minutes.

7. Then make a quick pressure release.

8. Let the cooked casserole rest for 10 minutes before serving.

Nutrition value/serving: calories 120, fat 7.9, fiber 0.9, carbs 7.5, protein 6.2

Almons and Mozzarella Zucchini Strips

Prep time: 10 minutes

Cooking time: 8 minutes

Servings: 2

Ingredients:

- 1 zucchini, trimmed

- 1/3 cup Mozzarella, shredded

- 1 teaspoon avocado oil

- 1 tablespoon almond meal

- ¼ teaspoon salt

Directions:

1. Cut the zucchini into the strips and sprinkle them with salt and almond meal.

2. Then heat up the instant pot on sauté mode for 2-3 minutes.

3. Add avocado oil.

4. Arrange the zucchini strips in one layer in the instant pot and cook them for 2 minutes from each side or until they are light brown.

5. Repeat the same steps with remaining zucchini strips (if you use small instant and can't arrange all vegetables per one time of cooking).

6. Then top the cooked zucchini strips with Mozzarella and close the lid.

7. Cook the side dish on sauté mode for 3 minutes or until the cheese is melted.

Nutrition value/serving: calories 49, fat 2.8, fiber 1.6, carbs 4.2, protein 3.2

Cabbage Rice

Prep time: 10 minutes

Cooking time: 35 minutes

Servings: 5

Ingredients:

- 1 ½ cup white cabbage, shredded

- 1 teaspoon salt

- 1 cup of coconut milk

- 1 teaspoon ground turmeric

- 1 white onion, diced

- 1 tablespoon coconut oil

Directions:

1. In the mixing bowl combine together salt and shredded cabbage. Leave the vegetables for 5 minutes.

2.   Meanwhile, heat up the instant pot bowl on sauté mode for 2 minutes.

3.   Add coconut oil and diced onion.

4.   Cook the onion for 3 minutes.

5.   Then stir it with the help of the spatula and add cabbage.

6.   After this, in the bowl combine together ground turmeric and coconut milk.

7.   When the liquid starts to be yellow, pour it over the cabbage.

8.   Stir the cabbage and close the lid.

9.   Cook the cabbage rice on sauté mode for 30 minutes. Stir ti from time to time to avoid burning.

Nutrition value/serving: calories 149, fat 14.2, fiber 2.2, carbs 6.2, protein 1.6

Cheddar Creamy Gratin

Prep time: 5 minutes

Cooking time: 7 minutes

Servings: 2

Ingredients:

- 1 cup turnip, sliced

- 1/3 cup heavy cream

- ¼ teaspoon salt

- ¼ teaspoon dried sage

- 1 teaspoon butter

- 1/3 teaspoon garlic powder

- ½ cup Cheddar cheese, shredded

Directions:

1. Toss butter in the instant pot and melt it on sauté mode (approx.2-3 minutes).

2.   Then add sliced turnip and cook it on sauté mode for 1 minute from each side.

3.   Sprinkle the vegetables with salt, dried sage, and garlic powder.

4.   Then add heavy cream.

5.   Top the turnip with Cheddar cheese and close the lid.

6.   Cook the meal on manual mode (high pressure) for 3 minutes. Then make a quick pressure release.

Nutrition value/serving: calories 220, fat 18.8, fiber 1.3, carbs 5.5, protein 8.1

White Onion Rings

Prep time: 10 minutes

Cooking time: 5 minutes

Servings: 4

Ingredients:

- 1 big white onion

- 1 egg, beaten

- 1 teaspoon cream cheese

- 2 oz Parmesan, grated

- 2 tablespoons almond meal

- 1 tablespoon butter

Directions:

1. Trim and peel the onion.

2. Then slice it roughly and separate every onion slice into the rings.

3.   In the mixing bowl combine together Parmesan and almond meal.

4.   Then take a separated bowl and mix up cream cheese and egg in it.

5.   Dip the onion rings in the egg mixture and then coat well in cheese mixture.

6.   Toss butter in the instant pot and melt it on sauté mode.

7.   Then arrange the onion rings in the melted butter in one layer.

8.   Cook the onion rings for 2 minutes from each side on sauté mode.

Nutrition value/serving: calories 122, fat 8.8, fiber 1.2, carbs 4.8, protein 7.1

Rosemary Halves

Prep time: 10 minutes

Cooking time: 10 minutes

Servings: 4

Ingredients:

- 3 cups radish, trimmed

- 1 tablespoon olive oil

- 1 teaspoon dried rosemary

- ½ teaspoon salt

Directions:

1. Cut the radishes into the halves and sprinkle with salt.

2. In the shallow bowl whisk together olive oil and dried rosemary.

3. After this, sprinkle the radish halves with fragrant oil and shake the vegetables well.

4. Transfer the radishes in the instant pot and cook the on sauté mode for 10 minutes.

5. Stir the vegetables every 2 minutes.

Nutrition value/serving: calories 45, fat 3.6, fiber 1.5, carbs 3.2, protein 0.6

Sweet Baby Carrot

Prep time: 10 minutes

Cooking time: 4 minutes

Servings: 4

Ingredients:

- 1 cup baby carrot

- 1 tablespoon Erythritol

- ½ teaspoon dried thyme

- 2 tablespoons butter, melted

- 1 cup water, for cooking

Directions:

1. Wash the baby carrot carefully and trim if needed.

2. Then pour water in the instant pot and insert the trivet,

3. Put the prepared baby carrots in the baking pan.

4.   Add dried thyme, Erythritol, and butter. Mix up the vegetables well and place over the trivet.

5.   Close the lid.

6.   Cook the carrot for 4 minutes on manual mode (high pressure).

7.   When the time is over make a quick pressure release.

Nutrition value/serving: calories 69, fat 5.8, fiber 1.1, carbs 7.8, protein 0.6

Chili Zucchini Bowl

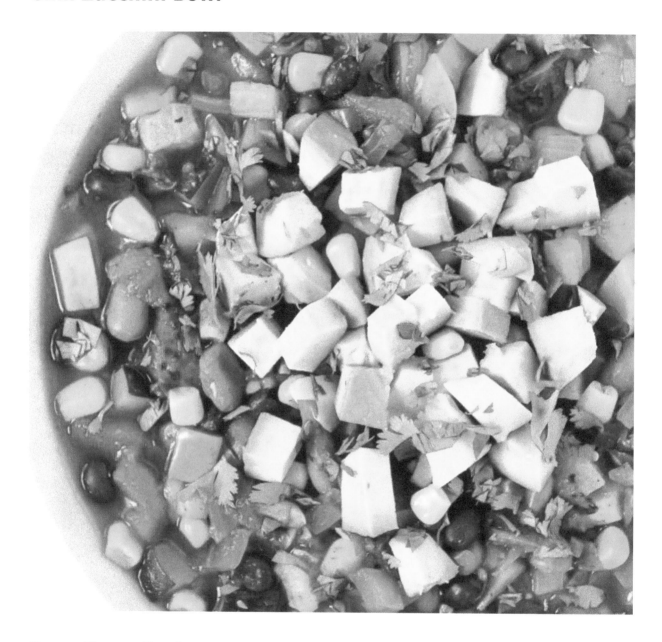

Prep time: 5 minutes

Cooking time: 3 minutes

Servings: 4

Ingredients:

- 2 zucchini, chopped

- 1 teaspoon olive oil

- ½ teaspoon chili flakes

- ½ teaspoon paprika

- 2 oz Feta, crumbled

Directions:

1. Place olive oil, zucchini, chili flakes, and paprika in the instant pot.

2. Stir the ingredients gently and close the lid.

3. Cook zucchini on sauté mode for 2 minutes.

4. Then open the lid and mix up them well with the help of the spatula.

5. Keep cooking zucchini for 1 minute more.

6. Transfer the cooked zucchini into the serving bowls and top with feta cheese.

Nutrition value/serving: calories 64, fat 4.4, fiber 1.2, carbs 4, protein 3.2

Thyme Asparagus

Prep time: 5 minutes

Cooking time: 5 minute

Servings: 2

Ingredients:

- 6 oz asparagus, trimmed

- ¼ teaspoon dried thyme

- ¼ teaspoon salt

- ¼ teaspoon ground black pepper

- ¼ teaspoon dried oregano

- ¼ teaspoon ground nutmeg

- 2 tablespoons butter

- ¼ cup chicken broth

Directions:

1.   In the mixing bowl combine together dried thyme, salt, ground black pepper, oregano, and nutmeg.

2.   Then put the asparagus in the instant pot.

3.   Sprinkle the vegetables with spice mixture. Stir them gently.

4.   Then add butter and chicken broth.

5.   Close the lid and cook asparagus on manual mode (high pressure) for 5 minutes.

6.   Then make the quick pressure release, open the lid, and shake the asparagus gently.

Nutrition value/serving: calories 127, fat 11.9, fiber 2.1, carbs 3.9, protein 2.7

Minced Radish

Prep time: 8 minutes

Cooking time: 3 minutes

Servings: 3

Ingredients:

- 1 ½ cup radish, sliced

- ½ teaspoon minced garlic

- 1 teaspoon sesame oil

- ¼ cup Monterey Jack cheese, shredded

- ¼ cup heavy cream

- 1 tablespoon cream cheese

Directions:

1.   Put radish minced garlic, sesame oil, heavy cream, and cream cheese in the instant pot.

2.   Mix up the radish mixture well.

3. Then top it with shredded cheese and close the lid.

4. Cook the radish for 3 minutes on Manual mode (high pressure).

5. Then make a quick pressure release.

Nutrition value/serving: calories 105, fat 9.3, fiber 0.9, carbs 2.6, protein 3.2

Peppery Cubes

Prep time: 10 minutes

Cooking time: 3 minutes

Servings: 6

Ingredients:

- 1-pound turnip, cubed

- 1 teaspoon salt

- ½ teaspoon ground black pepper

- 1 teaspoon avocado oil

- 1 cup water, for cooking

Directions:

1. Pour water and insert the steamer rack in the instant pot.

2. In the mixing bowl mix up together turnip cubes, salt, and ground black pepper.

3.   Sprinkle the vegetables with avocado oil and place them in the steamer rack.

4.   Close and seal the lid.

5.   Cook the turnip on Manual mode (high pressure) for 3 minutes.

6.   Then allow the natural pressure release for 5 minutes.

Nutrition value/serving: calories 23, fat 0.2, fiber 1.4, carbs 5, protein 0.7

Pecan Salad

Prep time: 10 minutes

Cooking time: 2 minutes

Servings: 2

Ingredients:

- 2 cups kale, chopped

- ½ cup fresh cilantro, chopped

- 1 pecan, chopped

- ½ teaspoon ground paprika

- ¼ teaspoon salt

- 1 tablespoon avocado oil

- 1 cucumber, chopped

- 1 cup water, for cooking

Directions:

1. Pour water and insert the steamer rack in the instant pot.

2. Place the kale in the steamer. Close and seal the lid.

3. Cook the greens for 2 minutes on Manual mode (high pressure).

4. Then make a quick pressure release and transfer the kale in the salad bowl.

5. Add chopped cilantro, pecan, and cucumber.

6. After this, sprinkle the salad with ground paprika, salt, and avocado oil.

7. Mix up the salad well.

Nutrition value/serving: calories 98, fat 6.2, fiber 3.1, carbs 9.2, protein 3

Cheese Gnocchi

Prep time: 15 minutes

Cooking time: 8 minutes

Servings: 6

Ingredients:

- 2 cups cauliflower, boiled

- 1 egg yolk

- ¼ cup coconut flour

- ½ cup almond meal

- 1 tablespoon cream cheese

- 2 oz Parmesan, grated

- 1 teaspoon dried basil

- 2 tablespoons butter

Directions:

1.   Place the boiled cauliflower in the food processor and blend it until smooth.

2.   Then add egg yolk, coconut flour, almond meal, cream cheese, and grated Parmesan.

3.   Blend the cauliflower mixture for 15 seconds more.

4.   Then transfer the mixture on the chopping board and knead it into the ball.

5.   Then cut the dough ball into 3 parts.

6.   After this, make 3 logs from the dough.

7.   Cut the logs into the small gnocchi with the help of the cutter.

8.   Toss the butter in the instant pot and melt it for 2 minutes on sauté mode.

9.   Add dried basil and bring the butter to boil (it will take around 1 minute).

10.   After this, add prepared gnocchi and cook them for 5 minutes. Stir the gnocchi from time to time.

Nutrition value/serving: calories 155, fat 11.7, fiber 3.8, carbs 7.3, protein 7.1

Purple Cabbage Steaks

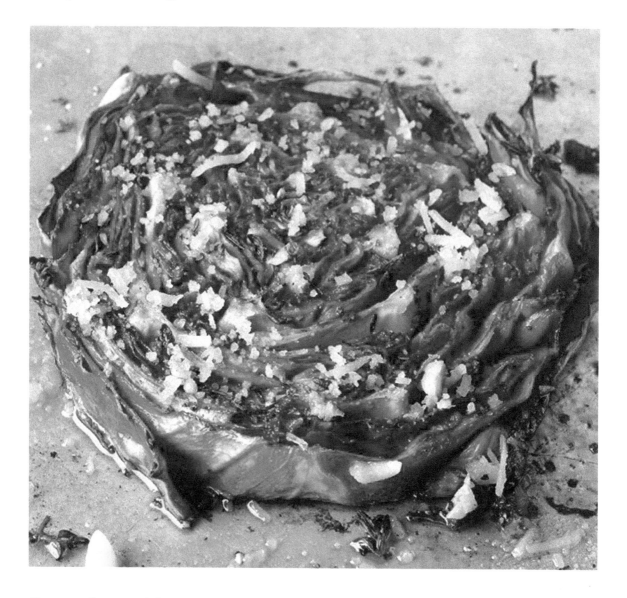

Prep time: 10 minutes

Cooking time: 4 minutes

Servings: 4

Ingredients:

- 10 oz purple cabbage

- 1 teaspoon apple cider vinegar

- 1 teaspoon olive oil

- ½ teaspoon salt

- ½ teaspoon lemon juice

- 1 cup water, for cooking

Directions:

1. Cut the purple cabbage into 4 cabbage steaks.

2. Pour water and insert the steamer rack in the instant pot.

3. Place the cabbage steaks on the rack and close the lid.

4. Cook the vegetables for 4 minutes on Manual mode (high pressure).

5. Then allow the natural pressure release for 5 minutes.

6. Place the cabbage steaks in the serving plates.

7.   In the shallow bowl whisk together apple cider vinegar, olive oil, salt, and lemon juice.

8.   Sprinkle every cabbage steak with apple cider vinegar mixture.

Nutrition value/serving: calories 28, fat 1.3, fiber 1.8, carbs 4.1, protein 0.9

Cauliflower and Goat Cheese

Prep time: 15 minutes

Cooking time: 5 minutes

Servings: 3

Ingredients:

- 1 ½ cup cauliflower, chopped

- ½ teaspoon salt

- 2 oz Goat cheese, crumbled

- 1 tablespoon cream cheese

- 1 cup water, for cooking

Directions:

1. Pour water and insert the steamer rack in the instant pot.

2. Place the cauliflower in the steamer rack and close the lid.

3. Cook the vegetables on manul mode (high pressure) for 5 minutes. Make a quick pressure release.

4. Place the cooked cauliflower in the food processor and blend it until smooth.

5. Transfer the cauliflower into the bowl. Add salt and cream cheese. Mix up the cauliflower mass well.

6. Place the cooked meal on the plate and top with goat cheese.

Nutrition value/serving: calories 110, fat 7.9, fiber 1.3, carbs 3.2, protein 7

Mushrooms and Fall Vegetables

Prep time: 10 minutes

Cooking time: 8 minutes

Servings: 5

Ingredients:

- 1 cup mushrooms, chopped

- 1 cup zucchini, chopped

- 1/2 cup bell pepper, chopped

- 1 eggplant, chopped

- 3 tablespoons butter

- ½ teaspoon salt

- 1 teaspoon dried basil

- 1 teaspoon dried thyme

- ½ teaspoon ground black pepper

- ½ teaspoon cayenne pepper

- 1 cup water, for cooking

Directions:

1. Pour water and insert the trivet in the instant pot.

2. Put all vegetables in the instant pot baking pan.

3. Sprinkle them with salt, dried basil, thyme, ground black pepper, and cayenne pepper.

4. Mix up the vegetables and top with butter.

5. Arrange the baking pan with vegetables in the instant pot.

6. Close the lid and cook the side dish for 8 minutes on Manual mode (high pressure).

7. Make a quick pressure release.

Nutrition value/serving: calories 96, fat 7.2, fiber 4, carbs 7.9, protein 1.9

Garlic Broccoli

Prep time: 10 minutes

Cooking time: 1 minute

Servings: 2

Ingredients:

- 1 cup broccoli florets

- ½ teaspoon garlic, diced

- ¼ teaspoon salt

- 1 teaspoon sesame oil

- 1 cup water, for cooking

Directions:

1. Pour water and insert the steamer rack in the instant pot.

2. Place the broccoli florets in the steamer rack and close the lid.

3. Cook the vegetables on Manual mode (high pressure) for 1 minute.

4. Then make a quick pressure release and transfer the cooked broccoli florets in the serving plates.

5. Sprinkle vegetables with garlic, salt, and sesame oil.

Nutrition value/serving: calories 37, fat 2.4, fiber 1.2, carbs 3.3, protein 1.3

Tots with Broccoli

Prep time: 10 minutes

Cooking time: 5 minutes

Servings: 4

Ingredients:

- 1 cup broccoli, shredded

- ¼ cup Cheddar cheese, shredded

- ¼ teaspoon garlic powder

- ¼ teaspoon salt

- 2 tablespoon almond meal

- ¼ teaspoon ground black pepper

- 1 teaspoon coconut oil

- 1 teaspoon dried dill

Directions:

1. In the mixing bowl combine together shredded broccoli, cheese, garlic powder, salt, almond meal, ground black pepper, and dried dill.

2. Mix up the mixture with the help of the spoon until homogenous.

3. After this, make the small tots from the mixture.

4. Heat up instant pot bowl on sauté mode for 3 minutes.

5. Then toss coconut oil and melt it (appx.1 minute).

6. Then arrange the tots in the instant pot in one layer and cook tots for 1 minute from each side.

Nutrition value/serving: calories 65, fat 5.1, fiber 1, carbs 2.6, protein 3.1

Vegetable Fritters

Prep time: 10 minutes

Cooking time: 6 minutes

Servings: 4

Ingredients:

- ½ cup turnip, boiled
- ½ cup cauliflower, boiled
- 1 egg, beaten
- 1 teaspoon dried parsley
- 3 tablespoons coconut flour
- 1 teaspoon avocado oil
- 1/3 teaspoon salt
- 1 teaspoon ground turmeric

Directions:

1.   Mash turnip and cauliflower with the help of the potato masher.

2.   Then add egg, dried parsley, coconut flour, salt, and ground turmeric in the mashed mixture and stir well.

3.   Make the medium side fritters and place them in the instant pot.

4.   Add avocado oil.

5.   Cook the fritters on sauté mode for 3 minutes from each side.

Nutrition value/serving: calories 50, fat 1.9, fiber 3, carbs 6, protein 2.6

Pressured Asparagus

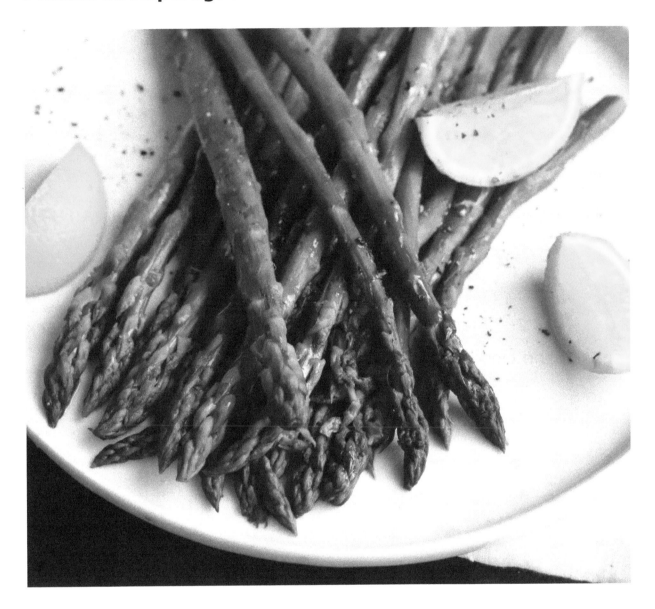

Prep time: 5 minutes

Cooking time: 1 minute

Servings: 2

Ingredients:

- 6 oz asparagus, chopped

- ¼ teaspoon salt

- 1 cup water, for cooking

Directions:

1. Pour water and insert the steamer rack in the instant pot.

2. Place the chopped asparagus in the steamer rack and close the lid.

3. Cook the vegetables on Manual (high pressure) for 1 minute.

4. Then make a quick pressure release and open the lid.

5. Sprinkle the asparagus with salt.

Nutrition value/serving: calories 17, fat 0.1, fiber 1.8, carbs 3.3, protein 1.9

Roasted Cider Steak

Prep time: 10 minutes

Cooking time: 4 minutes

Servings: 2

Ingredients:

- 8 oz cauliflower

- 1 teaspoon olive oil

- ½ teaspoon apple cider vinegar

- ¼ teaspoon chili flakes

- ¼ teaspoon salt

- ¼ teaspoon onion powder

- ¼ teaspoon ground turmeric

- 1 cup water, for cooking

Directions:

1.   Cut the cauliflower into medium steaks.

2.   In the shallow bowl combine together olive oil, apple cider vinegar, chili flakes, salt, onion powder, and ground turmeric.

3.   Then brush the cauliflower steaks with oily mixture form both sides.

4.   Pour water and insert the trivet in the instant pot.

5.   Arrange the cauliflower steaks in the instant pot in one layer.

6.   Cook the vegetables for 4 minutes on manual mode (high pressure).

7.   Then make a quick pressure release.

8.   Cool the cauliflower steaks for 2-5 minutes before serving.

Nutrition value/serving: calories 51, fat 2.5, fiber 2.9, carbs 6.5, protein 2.3

Cayenne Pepper Green Beans

Prep time: 10 minutes

Cooking time: 3 minutes

Servings: 4

Ingredients:

- 2 cups green beans, chopped

- 1 teaspoon cayenne pepper

- 1 tablespoon nut oil

- ¼ teaspoon salt

- 1 cup water, for coking

Directions:

1. Pour water and insert the steamer rack in the instant pot.

2. Place the green beans in the steamer rack.

3.   Cook the vegetables for 3 minutes on Manual mode (high pressure).

4.   Make a quick pressure release and cool the green beans in ice water for 4 minutes.

5.   Transfer the green beans in the mixing bowl and sprinkle with nut oil and salt. Mix up the beans well.

Nutrition value/serving: calories 48, fat 3.5, fiber 2, carbs 4.2, protein 1.1

Conclusion

Being a perfect solution both for instant pot novices and experienced split second pot customers this immediate pot recipe book raises your daily cooking. It makes you resemble a professional and also prepare like a pro. Thanks to the Instant Pot component, this recipe book assists you with preparing straightforward and tasty meals for any type of budget. Satisfy everybody with hearty dinners, nutritive breakfasts, sweetest treats, and also enjoyable snacks. Despite if you cook for one or prepare larger parts-- there's a solution for any possible food preparation circumstance. Improve your techniques on exactly how to cook in the most effective way using just your split second pot, this cookbook, and also some persistence to find out fast. Practical ideas as well as methods are discreetly incorporated right into every recipe to make your family demand new meals over and over again. Vegetarian choices, services for meat-eaters and also extremely satisfying suggestions to unify the entire family members at the same table. Consuming in your home is a common experience, and also it can be so good to satisfy all together at the end of the day. Master your Immediate Pot and also maximize this brand-new experience beginning today!

CPSIA information can be obtained
at www.ICGtesting.com
Printed in the USA
BVHW061433190521
607631BV00005B/873

9 781667 118639